D1711140

TABLE OF CONTENTS

LEGAL DISCLAIMER

The author and Healthy Kidney Publishing are legally obligated to include this disclaimer due to the litigious nature of today's world, which may give rise to accusations, criticisms and attempts to suppress and discredit the work.

This book or guide and all the information contained in it are copyrighted with all rights reserved. The author, the publisher and anyone associated or affiliated with Healthy Kidney Publishing do not assume any liability for the misuse or use of information contained herein.

The content in this guide or book is provided for educational and informational purposes only. It is not intended, nor should be a substitute for professional medical advice from a medical doctor, diagnoses or treatment. The author is not a medical doctor or a licensed health care professional, nor does he claim to be.

Never disregard professional medical advice from a licensed health care professional or delay in seeking it because of something you have read. Always consult your medical doctor or your primary health care provider about the application of any opinions or recommendations with respect to your own or someone else's symptoms or medical conditions.

Robert Galarowicz and Healthy Kidney Publishing and any of their websites, the author and anyone associated with them, shall have neither liability nor responsibility to any person or entity with respect to any loss, damage, or injury caused or alleged to be caused directly or indirectly by the information contained in this guide.

Every attempt has been made to provide information that is both accurate and proven effective; the author, Healthy Kidney Publishing and by extension the guide or book, make no guarantees that the remedies, nutrition, diet, supplements, testing, lifestyle changes and any information presented herein will help everyone in every situation. As the symptoms, diseases and/or conditions for each person are unique to the individual histories, body type, physical conditioning, medical conditions, and the specifics of the actual kidney disease, success will vary.

You should never stop taking any medication without first consulting with your medical doctor or health care provider. You should consult with your medical doctor or health care provider before beginning any health maintenance or health improvement program.

All information contained and any links are for informational purposes only and are not warranted for content, accuracy or any other implied or explicit purposes.

This guide or book is sold subject to the condition that it shall not by way of trade or otherwise, be rented, lent, sold, hired out, given away or otherwise distributed without the author or publisher's consent.

Not one single part of this book, guide, and publication may be reproduced, edited, stored in a system or transmitted in any form or by any means. No transmission by electronic, mechanical including photocopying, digital, recorded or otherwise, without the prior written consent of the author or publisher.

This book and guide is based on discoveries made by researchers in the United States and Worldwide. It is rooted from the expertise of medical journals, scientific papers, medical reports, books, and other manuscripts.

This is NOT a free book or guide. So, you do not have the right to resell it.

Copyright 2020 © Healthy Kidney Publishing

ISBN: 9798662666610

THE COMPLETE GUIDE TO SUPPLEMENTS FOR KIDNEY HEALTH INTRODUCTION

"The 'Just Get Me Started' Version" – If you are going through the later stages of kidney disease such as stages 3, 4 or 5. You should reference Chapter 8:The Core Natural Kidney Health Supplements Explained & Product Recommendations and Chapter 9: Stage 4 & 5 Kidney Disease & Avoiding Dialysis.

This book is dedicated to anyone who is suffering from kidney disease and may have even been told by their doctors:

"There is nothing you can do, you have to wait for your kidneys to fail, go on dialysis and hopefully be eligible for a kidney transplant."

Now you have options …

I have been through every phase of chronic kidney disease including dialysis and have undergone a cadaver kidney transplant. This book is the culmination of a life's work to help you avoid what I've been through.

The field of kidney disease (medical term "nephrology") is in its infancy. We are just beginning to get a grasp on how the kidney fully functions and the effects that lifestyles, environment, nutrition and diseases have on the organs.

Until about 1970, kidney failure meant absolute death. Once your kidneys could no longer function, it was just a matter of time until you passed away. An even more alarming fact is that until 2002, no standard definition for chronic kidney disease (CKD) existed within the medical community.

This means the medical community, researchers and doctors didn't fully have chronic kidney disease properly categorized. It took time for everyone to agree to standards. Once this was done, it emerged that an epidemic of kidney disease was upon America and in fact the world.

In the last 30 to 50 years (a small time within the health field) medical systems from different countries have researched and developed their own methods for treating chronic kidney disease.

For the most part, many of these methods aren't used in the U.S. and foreign countries, even though in parts of Europe, South America and the South Pacific some methods are considered standard, and insurance and pharmaceutical companies cover and manufacture these natural therapies.

Why is this?

Until the widespread use of the internet, the world didn't have the capacity to easily share accurate medical information that was substantiated by reputable research. Now that we are able to easily share that information, anything considered valuable has to be funded and rigorously tested through each country's medical system before it can be incorporated into standard care.

This is regardless of the substances being used safely in countries for 30+ years. Each medical system has its own process that needs to be followed to protect their public. This process is slowed down or stopped by enormous amounts of unexpected problems.

For example, when the United States' National Institute of Health wanted to study rhubarb, a Chinese herbal medication for kidney disease, they couldn't find or keep enough people in the study, due to various reasons so they had to discontinue it.

This process is also halted by very high financing costs -- a modern day pharmaceutical drug can cost $200 million before it reaches the public – as well as bureaucratic paperwork, special interest groups and many unexpected issues.

Treatments have been discovered for kidney disease and other diseases, but it can take 25 years to complete the process of discovery to standard care and bring it to the point where it can help the public.

Aside from medications and supplements, diet is critical to the health of your kidneys. Therapeutic diets for kidney health is beyond the scope of this book. For dietary recommendations see our book called, "The Complete Guide To Renal Diet Plans &

Cook Books" available on Amazon.

If you have questions, comments, a success story or anything you feel I should add to the guide, send me an email at: healthykidneyinc@gmail.com.

Sincerely,

Robert Galarowicz

CHAPTER 1 THE KIDNEYS AND THEIR FUNCTION

The kidney is an amazing organ, only about 4 ½ inches in length, weighing about 6 ounces. Its functions are many and vital to our body's health and wellness, and how lucky we are to have two of them.

They can be found in the abdomen, under the ribs, and while responsible for regulating many of the body's necessary functions, their main purpose is to filter and remove waste products from the body.

It also keeps a proper balance of the blood plasma's contents, i.e., salts, potassium, acid, and other important components. These components make up the extracellular fluid where millions of our cells live and do their job, and which are circulated by the blood system throughout the body.

Other functions of the kidneys include:

- Balancing the body's fluids, including making urine

- Releasing hormones that regulate blood pressure

- Removing drugs and some toxins from the body

- Producing an active form of vitamin D that promotes strong, healthy bones

- Controlling the production of red blood cells

- Maintaining acid-alkaline balance (PH level), *aka*, acid-base balance

- Producing L-Carnitine, a substance that helps the body turn fat into energy, and which, if lacking, can often contribute to fatigue in kidney disease.

The kidneys possess remarkable and complex mechanisms to get all this work done.

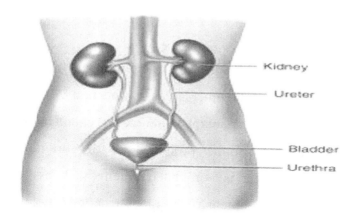

Figure 1.1 Front View of the Kidneys

From the kidneys, the ureters conduct urine to the bladder,

which empties out of the body through the urethra.

Within each kidney lies the glomerulus, or tiny blood vessels.

Liquid from the blood plasma collects here. This liquid has already been filtered by the glomerular membrane, and the protein molecules have already been removed.

Now called the glomerular filtrate, the liquid passes down a small but long tube or *tubule* and reaches a pouch called the kidney pelvis; eventually the liquid drains into the urethra. During the journey, the components in the liquid have been reabsorbed with some secretions added. What's left is urine.

Though the popular belief is that the kidney's function is to excrete wastes, as you can see, they play a much bigger role than that. Much like the lungs, which most people believe simply take in oxygen, when in actuality, they also simultaneously release carbon dioxide.

Hormones play a big part of helping the kidneys. Certain hormones, produced in other areas of the body, are sent to the kidneys by the blood plasma, and act like a "chemical messenger." For example, a hormone produced in the brain, called the antidiuretic hormone, is stimulated when the body loses water when in a hot environment. The kidney responds by lessening the volume of urine enabling the body to hold on to more water. On the other hand, after drinking a large amount of water, this hormone is "turned off" and the kidneys go back to excreting more urine.

For those who can't make the antidiuretic hormone, or whose

kidneys don't respond to it (known as diabetes insipidus – no relation to type 1 or type 2 diabetes), the kidneys will excrete large amounts of urine and remain thirsty. Their water intake is equal with their urine output and remains in a slightly dehydrated state.

The kidneys produce not only their own hormones (an important vitamin), but are also involved with production of an amino acid. Below is a listing of hormones that the kidneys produce:

- Angiotensin: raises blood pressure by constricting blood vessels, and acts as a stimulator to create another hormone, called "aldosterone," which regulates the excretion of sodium.

- Erythropoietin: stimulates bone marrow to produce more red cells when needed. (Explains why anemia is a common symptom of kidney disease.)

- Prostaglandins: helps regulate blood pressure, inflammation and the excretion of sodium among other functions.

- Vitamin D: Also considered a vitamin and a hormone, and is necessary for the proper circulation of calcium and phosphorous, which is vital for healthy bones. (A deficiency in vitamin D is also a symptom of kidney failure.)

The kidneys are the great multitaskers of the body, making it easy to understand that when they do malfunction certain death can occur in just a few weeks. However, rest assured that since we are fortunate to have two of them, even if they lose even 90% of their functioning, with proper care, the otherwise healthy individual will survive.

CHAPTER 2 KIDNEY DISEASE, ITS STAGES AND SYMPTOMS

A loss of kidney function is called kidney disease. It is often referred to as "chronic kidney disease" (CKD). Kidney failure is the final stage of CKD when the organs are only operating at 15% or less of their potential.

At that point, kidney failure is then divided into two categories:

- Chronic kidney failure. When your kidneys have gradually lost function over time and are no longer able to handle their function within the body. At this point, dialysis or a kidney transplant is needed.

- Acute kidney failure. When urine output is drastically reduced and the kidneys begin to accumulate waste products. Dialysis may be required, and patients can recover with proper care. Causes of acute kidney failure include drugs that are toxic to the organs, surgical complications, i.e., severe reduction in blood flow among others.

The 5 Stages of Kidney Disease

There are five stages of kidney disease, numbered 1 through 5, each representing a level of the organ's functioning. Mild cases would be numbered one and two; moderate is number three; and advanced are four and five. Once kidney disease has been diagnosed, it's vital to understand the differences in each of these five stages.

The formula used to determine at what stage your kidneys are still functioning as filters is called the GFR, or *glomerular filtration rate*, and is measured in *milliliters per minute* (ml/min). Become familiar with the GFR, as this measurement is what is used to monitor your kidney disease. Normal GFR is the range between 100 to 130 ml/min.

Stage 1

Kidney function is normal, or near normal; the kidneys are working around 90 percent, with possible *proteinuria* present, meaning that protein is present in the urine.

Proteinuria is a very important factor in kidney disease. The amount of protein in urine is the most important predictor for worsening kidney function.

In stage 1, GFR is around 90 ml/min. If left untreated, the condition of the kidneys can worsen. A consultation with a medical doctor who specializes in kidney disease (nephrologist) is usually in order, and active measures to prevent further decline should be taken.

Stage 2

A further decline in kidney functioning with a GFR of around 60 to 89 ml/min is considered stage 2 kidney disease. Protein in the urine may or may not be present, but close monitoring of the kidneys is crucial.

Stage 3

GFR is around 30 to 59 ml/min. In stages 1 and 2, other systems in the body aren't yet affected, but in stage 3, changes in blood and bone health will be seen.

This stage is broken up into two. Stage 3a which is a decrease in glomerular filtration rate (GFR) between 45-59 mL/min. Stage 3b is a decrease in GFR for 30-44 mL/min.

Stage 4

Signs of advanced kidney disease are being seen, and a GFR of 15 to 29 is present. At this time, the person may develop complications like high blood pressure, anemia (a shortage of red blood cells), bone disease and heart disease.

Stage 5

A person with stage 5 CKD has end-stage renal disease (ESRD) with a GFR of 15 ml/min or less. At this advanced stage of kidney disease, the kidneys have lost nearly all their ability to do their job effectively, and eventually dialysis or a kidney transplant will be needed for survival. At this stage, a very aggressive approach should be taken. In many cases, an improvement in function or delay in dialysis has occurred with my program.

Symptoms of Kidney Disease

Sometimes symptoms of kidney disease do not present until a significant loss of kidney function is seen, sometimes even in the 3rd or 4th stage.

The most common symptoms are fatigue, muscle cramps, loss of appetite, nausea, problems with urination, edema (swelling mostly in the ankles and legs, but can occur in other parts of the body), vomiting, easy bruising, depression, itching and shortness of breath.

Other less common symptoms are thirst, headache, a bad taste in the mouth, insomnia, twitching or restless legs, difficulty concentrating, impaired memory, numbness and tingling in the hands and feet, urinating frequently especially at night, diarrhea or constipation.

CHAPTER 3 EVALUATING AND TESTING FOR KIDNEY DISEASE

How Tests Confirm Kidney Disease?

If kidney disease is suspected, there are a host of tests that can determine the level of kidney functioning; a kidney specialist or nephrologist may order a few different tests since what one may miss, another test will pick up. Unfortunately, kidney disease can be present in people that have little or no complaints and those over 50 years of age should include a kidney analysis as part of their routine health checkups.

Urine Tests

The Glomerular Filtration Rate (GFR), as mentioned before, assesses the rate and capacity of the kidney filtering process. A healthy male will have a GFR range of between 100-130 ml/min. and for a healthy female that number falls to 90-115 ml/min. As kidney disease progresses, the GFR number falls below 90 and may continue to fall.

A urinalysis is the basic test used to pre-screen kidney disease. Even if the GFR is normal, this test can pick up abnormalities quickly and effortlessly.

What is checked is proteinuria and a urinary protein called albumin. If there is presence of albumin in the urine or albuminuria, further urine testing will be ordered.

The urine test will also check the presence of a urinary tract infection as well as glucose which could indicate diabetes; the presence of blood can be a sign that kidney inflammation is present.

24 Hour Urine Test

A 24 hour urine test is more conclusive than a urinalysis, and requires that the urine be continuously collected for 24 hours. This requires urinating into a special plastic container every time you need to void. This is a more quantitative test that shows the amount of protein present in the urine.

In a healthy person, up to 150 milligrams (mg) of protein can be eliminated daily in urine. Greater amount of protein in urine is called proteinuria.

As discussed earlier, proteinuria can be an early sign of kidney disease. The amount of protein in urine is the most important predictor for worsening kidney function.

Self-Testing for Kidney Disease

One easy way to self-test and monitor your kidney disease is to check for protein in the urine.

Protein in the urine can be detected by paper test strips called Uri strips. These strips are available without prescription and can be found at a local pharmacy or online. To test, hold Uri strip in a urinary stream and follow instructions on a package for a color change. A change in color may indicate protein or glucose in the urine. Presence of protein or glucose in the urine, not previously seen, needs to be reported to your doctor.

Note: a temporary presence of protein in the urine can also be caused by vigorous exercise, infection, fever, or very high blood sugar. Repeat the test on a different day to check for persistent presence of protein or glucose in the urine.

Notify your doctor if protein or glucose is repeatedly present in the urine. If the color of the Uri strip does not change, neither protein nor glucose is present in the urine.

However, if you are at risk or have kidney disease, or diabetes, you should test frequently for the presence of protein or glucose in the urine.

Blood Tests

Creatinine is a material produced in the muscles and filtered by the kidneys. A blood test can provide a "creatinine number" to help indicate kidney function. The lower the number, the better the kidneys are performing.

However, many factors can influence the creatinine number like the person's muscle size and medications being taken at the time of the test.

One of the most widely used blood tests, the BUN (Blood Urea Nitrogen) test, is often used in tandem with the creatinine level, which can alert doctors to improperly functioning kidneys. If the BUN level is very high, then dehydration may be present. However, this condition may also be caused by other health conditions such as heart problems or diabetes. Abnormal levels of electrolytes like sodium bicarbonate, potassium, and phosphorus in the blood can also be an indicator.

Blood pH is another level that can be thrown off balance by kidney disease.

When kidney disease is present, anemia can set in, so red blood cell counts should be checked including hemoglobin and hematocrit. One of the hormones the kidneys produce is the blood-building hormone erythropoietin which declines as kidney disease worsens. Erythropoietin levels should also be tested.

There are additional tests you doctor will order to check for anemia such as serum ferritin, serum iron, transferring, transferring saturation, TIBC (total iron binding capacity) and UIBC (unsaturated iron binding capacity).

Albumin is the main protein in the blood, malnutrition and kidney disease can cause the levels of this protein to go down. This is monitored in the blood to check your protein nutrition status.

L-Carnitine is an amino acid that is largely made by the kidney and low levels and deficiencies can contribute to anemia, fatigue and increased kidney damage. The majority of medical doctors don't test for this, but it is something that you should ask for to determine if you need supplementation.

A uric acid test measures the amount of uric acid in the blood. Uric acid is produced from the natural breakdown of the foods you eat. Uric acid is mostly filtered out by the kidneys and leaves the body through urine. If the kidneys are not able to remove it from the body, the level of uric acid in the blood increases.

High levels of uric acid cause a painful condition within joints called gout and also can cause kidney stones or kidney failure. It's very important to get tested for uric acid and be treated if you have high levels.

Ultrasound, Cat Scans and MRI's

Once the blood work is completed and evidence of kidney disease is present, an ultrasound is probably the next step. By obtaining a visual picture of the kidneys, your physician can see the kidney size and texture, and it will help to determine if there are kidney stones present, or if there are signs of chronic kidney disease.

CAT scans and MRI's may also be ordered, but they do not come risk-free. This is addressed in greater detail on page 63.

Kidney Biopsy

Lastly, taking a biopsy and analyzing a small tissue sample of the kidney may help determine the cause of the kidney disease.

Heavy Metal Testing

Pollution can also cause kidney damage. Heavy metals such as lead, cadmium, uranium, mercury, arsenic and others are found to contribute to or cause kidney disease. I would highly recommend asking your medical doctor for a heavy metal test.

Autoimmune Diseases

Autoimmune diseases are when your immune system attacks healthy cells in your body by mistake. Autoimmune diseases can affect many parts of the body, including the kidney.

Your doctor will check you for autoimmune kidney diseases. However, it is recommended to check for all autoimmune diseases as there have been cases of autoimmune diseases not originally thought to effect the kidney, that actually have.

Celiac Disease

Celiac disease is an autoimmune disorder that can occur in genetically predisposed people where eating gluten leads to damage in the small intestine, causing a variety of symptoms. There is also a high correlation with celiac disease and kidney disease. There are many cases of kidney disease stemming from undiagnosed celiac disease. Therefore, it is recommended you are checked for this.

Other Testing

There are other tests (not used very often, however) that your doctor may perform such as Cystatin C, interleukins, and cytokines.

CHAPTER 4 WHAT CAUSES KIDNEY DISEASE?

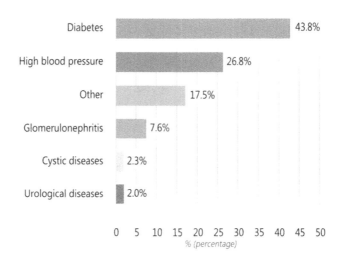

Source: United States Renal Data System. USRDS 2014 Annual Data Report.

Causes of Chronic Kidney Disease (CKD)

The two most common medical conditions responsible for causing CKD are diabetes and hypertension. Ironically, diabetes and hypertension are also the most preventable causes of kidney disease through lifestyle changes including weight loss, exercise, supplements and dietary modifications.

Diabetes

Diabetes Mellitus, commonly known as diabetes, is a multi-organ damaging medical condition that can affect the eyes, nerves, nervous system, blood vessels, heart, and the kidneys.

There are two types of diabetes: type 1 and type 2. In type 1 diabetes, the body stops making insulin. In most cases, type 1 diabetes is diagnosed at a young age. In type 2 diabetes, the body makes insulin, but the insulin does not function properly or the body becomes resistant to its own insulin due to obesity and other conditions.

When diabetes leads to kidney disease, it is called diabetic nephropathy. Diabetic nephropathy is the most common cause of CKD in the U.S. due to the rapid rise of the number of people diagnosed with diabetes.

How Diabetes Affects the Kidneys

Diabetes is the number one cause of chronic kidney disease accounting for nearly half or 43.8% of chronic kidney disease diagnoses. High blood sugar (glucose) levels in the blood increase stress and workload on the kidneys.

High blood sugar levels can affect the integrity of blood vessels within the kidneys making the blood vessels become narrow and clogged, and eventually cut off circulation (blood supply) to the kidneys leading to chronic kidney disease.

High blood sugar levels can cause damage to blood vessels in the entire body, including the heart. In addition, high blood sugar levels cause inflammation to the blood vessels within the kidneys and form scar tissue, further worsening kidney function.

High blood sugar can cause damage to the nerve supply in the entire body, including the kidneys and the bladder. The bladder muscles become weaker, and when the kidneys excrete (eliminate) urine to the bladder, the urine accumulates within the bladder. When the bladder is full, pressure builds up in the kidneys causing them to work harder adding stress, which in turn may worsen the kidney function.

High sugar levels in the blood increase the chances of developing frequent, chronic and/or difficult to treat urinary tract infections, since bacteria favors a sugar environment.

Since nerve supply is affected by those with diabetes, they may not even know they have a urinary tract infection; if left untreated, the bacteria can travel up and spread infection to the kidneys, which can worsen kidney function.

Hypertension

Hypertension, or high blood pressure, is a silent killer since most people do not experience any symptoms. Hypertension affects many organs of the body including the heart, the brain, blood vessels, and the kidneys.

A blood pressure reading consists of two numbers: the top number (or the one mentioned first) is the systolic blood pressure. The bottom number, or second one mentioned, is called diastolic blood pressure.

As a part of the aging process, the systolic blood pressure (the top number) generally increases with age. When it comes to monitoring blood pressure, both numbers require attention, as blood pressure increases the risk of heart disease, stroke, and kidney disease.

Hypertension is diagnosed on a basis of several measurements taken over time. A single blood pressure reading does not confirm a diagnosis of hypertension since blood pressure is affected by physical, emotional, and pharmacologic (such as caffeine) factors.

A normal blood pressure is defined as a systolic blood pressure (the top number) of 120 or less, and/or diastolic blood pressure (the bottom number) of 80 or less.

There are different stages of hypertension, depending on the blood pressure level. Prehypertension is defined as a systolic blood pressure of 120 to 139 and/or a diastolic blood pressure of 80 to 89. In this stage, it is very important to adopt lifestyle changes to prevent the development of hypertension.

Stage 1 hypertension is defined as a systolic blood pressure of 140 to 159 and/or diastolic blood pressure of 90 to 99. Stage 2 hypertension is defined as a systolic blood pressure of 160 or higher and/or diastolic blood pressure of 100 or higher.

A rapid elevation of blood pressure at a doctor's office in a presence of normal blood pressure readings at home is termed "white-coat syndrome."

How Hypertension Affects the Kidneys

Hypertension is the second most common cause of kidney disease in the US and the leading cause among African-Americans.

The kidneys are structured to handle blood pressure in a range of 130/80. If the blood pressure and the pressure delivered to the kidneys remain high over an extended period of time, it causes harmful effects to the function of the kidneys.

If the blood pressure is high, the pressure to the kidneys is high. The pressure at which kidneys need to filter blood is also high. This makes the kidneys work harder putting them at a high risk of stress, which can lead to CKD.

High blood pressure also causes inflammatory changes to the blood vessels of the kidneys. Over time, prolonged high blood pressure causes scarring of the arteries in the kidneys. If left untreated, hypertension can lead to irreversible scarring (fibrosis) to the kidneys and development of CKD.

Glomerulonephritis

In addition to diabetes and hypertension, high levels of

inflammation and inflammatory conditions can cause kidney disease.

Glomerulonephritis is an inflammation of the glomeruli of the kidneys. Glomerulus is a set of very small blood vessels within the kidneys forming a complex filtering system that cleans the blood of excess minerals in order to keep the body in balance. The kidneys are composed of millions of glomeruli.

In glomerulonephritis, the degree of inflammation can range from very mild to severe. Depending on what kind of infection or condition is causing the glomerulonephritis, more than one body system can be affected like in lupus and rheumatoid arthritis.

Glomerulonephritis includes a large list of conditions and disorders with varying causes, presentations, and outcomes. The most common causes of glomerulonephritis are IgA nephropathy (Berger's disease) and post-streptococcal glomerulonephritis.

IgA is a protein that acts as an antibody which helps fight infections. IgA nephropathy occurs when too much of this protein deposits in the glomeruli of the kidneys. Buildup of IgA in the glomeruli causes inflammation and damage to the glomeruli. The disorder can develop suddenly (called acute glomerulonephritis) or can develop slowly over many years (called chronic glomerulonephritis).

Post-streptococcal glomerulonephritis can occur several weeks after a strep throat infection. Post-streptococcal glomerulonephritis predominates in children and young adults and it usually gets better on its own after several weeks.

Polycystic Kidney Disease

The most common of the cystic diseases that causes chronic kidney disease is Polycystic Kidney Disease (PKD). When multiple cysts are discovered on the kidneys, a diagnosis of polycystic kidney disease, or ADPKD, can be made. ADPKD stands for autosomal dominant polycystic kidney disease which is an inherited condition. It is passed down from generation to generation and a family member has a 50% chance of developing it. There have been cases where a sudden appearance of the cysts occurred in a patient without having an inflicted parent or other relative.

The condition can be divided into two types: the more aggressive PKD1 where the disease progresses quickly into the end stage or PKD2 where the disease moves slower.

These cysts, or fluid-filled sacs, can grow large enough to actually overtake the kidney, compressing and squeezing it, and as the cysts continue to grow, high blood pressure usually results. Cysts can become so enlarged that they are visible from outside the body. In some cases, the disease can cause cysts to grow on the liver, which is not always problematic, but as the disease progresses, brain aneurysms can occur causing very serious bleeding, requiring surgery to correct.

DNA testing can be done on infants that can determine if the condition is present, but it can be expensive and not always conclusive or easy to understand. Years later, when the child reaches their 20's is when a more definitive test, usually an ultrasound, might be ordered to detect any sign of the disease. The disease may not be seen until even the 30's and beyond.

Urological Disease or Kidney Blockage

The kidneys, as mentioned earlier, are attached to tubes or ureters and the fluid is sent to the bladder. When full, the bladder's reflex is to empty itself. The urine than flows through a smaller tube called the urethra. The urethra carries the urine out of the body.

These three parts of the body: kidneys, ureters and bladder form the urinary tract. If a blockage is present in the ureters, the release of urine is stalled and backs up in the kidneys. It may distort the shape of the organ and most likely affect its ability to function. This is called hydronephrosis.

When complete urinary tract obstruction occurs, it is extremely dangerous and acute renal failure can result. As men age, 55 and over in most cases, they may suffer difficulties in urination, usually caused by an enlarged prostate. This is called benign prostatic hyperplasia (BPH).

Symptoms of BPH include frequent urination, difficulty in initiating urination, and having to urinate often during the night. A urologist will order an ultrasound of the kidneys and bladder if this is suspected. Surgery can relieve the obstruction, and in most cases, the kidneys will recover if the problem is diagnosed early. If the obstruction is present for a prolonged period of time, significant loss of kidney function can occur. In some cases, this can lead to kidney failure.

Other Causes of Chronic Kidney Disease

Other causes of chronic kidney disease can include: potassium deficiency, pollution, acute or chronic dehydration, chronic use of pain killers, chronic lithium use, Alport's syndrome, auto-immune diseases like lupus, severe dehydration, connective tissue disease, kidney stones, hardening of the arteries (vascular disease), heavy metal toxicity, infections, certain cancers, HIV Infection, heroin abuse, ischemic nephropathy, amyloidosis, poor lifestyle habits (bad diet, sedentary lifestyle, smoking, alcohol abuse, etc), liver cirrhosis and complement syndromes.

A Special Note on Obesity and how it Affects the Kidneys

A special note should be made about obesity since it has reached epidemic proportions in the U.S. with an estimated 30% of the population considered obese.

Obesity is defined as a body mass index (BMI) of 30 or greater. BMI is a calculation of body weight divided by height then squared.

Excess weight creates damaging effects to our health and our body. Excess weight places more stress on the kidneys making the kidneys work harder.

In addition, obesity leads to high blood pressure (hypertension), sleep apnea, insulin resistance, high cholesterol, and proteinuria, even in absence of diabetes. And, while hypertension, diabetes, and obesity are separate conditions, they often occur together.

CHAPTER 5 INFLAMMATION AND OXIDATIVE STRESS IN KIDNEY DISEASE

Inflammation in the kidneys can create and worsen kidney function. And while the role that inflammation has in kidney function, or dysfunction, is still being studied by scientists and physicians, there are four areas of concern:

1. That when chronic kidney disease (CKD) is present, there is inflammation seen as well.

2. Some main causes of chronic kidney disease such as hypertension and diabetes cause inflammation.

3. Obesity which is often seen in combination with diabetes and hypertension is now considered a state of inflammation.

4. Other organs can be affected by an inflammation of the kidneys, especially the heart.

Therefore, preventing and reducing inflammation is a key factor in treating kidney disease.

What is Inflammation and How Does it Start?

Inflammation is a body's response to any type of illness, disease, or trauma. Even a small cut in a skin sets off an inflammatory response. The body starts producing special proteins called cytokines that begin the healing process.

When damage happens inside the cells of the body, inflammatory response is also activated. Damaged cells start producing toxic substances called free radicals. In contrary, healthy cells start producing antioxidants to offset toxic free radicals to maintain balance at the cellular level.

If the damage to the cells continues for a prolonged period of time or is severe enough, excessive amounts of free radicals are produced. Cellular injury induced by excess of freeradicals is called oxidative stress. Oxidative stress occurs when production of toxic free radicals exceeds the production of antioxidants.

Excess amounts of free radicals stimulate the production of cytokines. Many cytokines cause chronic inflammatory changes, including production of scar tissue at a cellular level.

Chronic kidney disease (CKD) is an inflammatory condition. CKD itself can cause oxidative stress and further stimulate inflammatory response. This can lead to scarring of the kidneys leading to more inflammation, creating a vicious, never-ending cycle.

And, since CKD is an inflammatory condition in itself, the inflammatory response process is never turned off. Thus, it is very important to treat inflammation and free radical damage, as well as other conditions of kidney disease such as hypertension or diabetes, to preserve kidney function.

CHAPTER 6 UREMIA AND CHRONIC KIDNEY DISEASE

Uremic syndrome (uremia) is a complication of chronic kidney disease and renal failure. It occurs when urea and other waste products (kidney toxins) such as d-amino acids, peptides and proteins, guanidines, phenols, other aromatic compounds, indoles and other tryptophan metabolites, advanced glycation end products, aliphatic amines, etc., and other substances build up in the body, because the kidneys are unable to eliminate them.

These substances can become poisonous (toxic) to the body if they reach high levels and further damage the kidney causing a loss of kidney function.

Parts of the uremic toxins are generated in the intestine and can become deposited in the intestines from the blood. Many of the toxins created or deposited in the intestines play an active role in vascular and kidney damage and a disruption in the intestinal flora, accelerating the loss of kidney function.

Intestinal flora are living organisms that live within the intestinal tract of humans and animals. This flora is called probiotics and when introduced in high numbers has beneficial effects on the host and especially in kidney disease.

Probiotics are beneficial "good" bacteria that break down uremic toxins, synthesize vitamins, boost the immune system, defend against infections and perform other health benefits. In kidney disease, probiotics become altered and decreased, which can lead to an increase in inflammation and a reduction in effective elimination of uremic toxins.Probiotics will be discussed further in Chapter 7.

Probiotics have been studied in human trials, and have been shown to improve kidney function, digestive problems, immune system, other issues, and quality of life. Probiotics are very important to support normal kidney function.

Fiber supplements are another product that will improve kidney function by decreasing the amount of uremic toxin buildup and removing the toxins from the body. There have been various fiber supplements studied, but the preferred fiber supplement to decrease proteinuria is discussed in Chapter 7.

This field of kidney disease is rarely discussed in western medical treatments. It is also referred to as "Intestinal NitrogenRecycling, Urea Nitrogen Recycling and Intestinal Therapeutic Interventions," this aspect of kidney disease has been studied more in other countries.

However, In the last ten years there are more studies supporting their use in Western Medicine Literature. The therapies help decrease uremic toxin buildup thereby slowing or halting chronic kidney disease. I have seen many positive benefits when high doses of probiotics, high dose acacia fiber and diet are used to support kidney health.

CHAPTER 7 THE COMPLETE GUIDE TO SUPPLEMENTS FOR KIDNEY HEALTH CORE SUPPLEMENTS

In this Chapter, we will cover the "Core Supplements." These are the core supplements for supporting normal kidney function.

Regardless of the type of kidney disease, the core supplements are meant to be taken. However, this is on a case-by-case basis.

Ideally, everyone should take all the supplements recommended, have the perfect diet and take all their medications. This is often not realistic for most people due to lifestyle, finances, and personal preferences.

If you find taking the core supplements in addition to any supplements recommended for your condition overwhelming and not feasible, then choose the supplements for your specific kidney disease, and you can add in any additional ones you desire. Also, take advantage of your 60 days of email support if you need any assistance or clarification.

Following chapters will cover additional supplements for specific kidney diseases and kidney-related ailments.Regardless of what supplement you purchase, all supplements are to be taken with food or meals unless otherwise noted.

Each supplement mentioned will have a listing of quality-controlled manufacturers, specific products and appropriate quantities.

If you decide to use brands other than those listed here, you MUST use the same doses as the products recommended.

The products recommended and doses are what have been shown in research to benefit kidney disease. If you do not use the same therapeutic doses, you will not get the improvement you are looking for.

The Core Program Supplement Overview

(Each supplement is explained in the following pages)

- **Multivitamin** 1 to 2 pills per day with food.

- **Fish Oil** EPA 1500 to 5000mg and DHA 1000 to 4000mg per day in two or three divided doses with food.

- **Vitamin D3 (Cholecalciferol - if needed)** 2,000 to 5,000IUs once per day with food.

- **Sodium Bicarbonate (if needed)** ½ tablet (325mg) to 1 tablet (650mg) per day between meals/empty stomach to start.

- **Probiotics** 60-100 billion CFUs per day or more between meals or with food. Probiotic products should contain the strains Lactobacillus acidophilus, and Bifidobacterium longum. Any additional strains added are okay to take.

- **"Probiotic Loading"** The first 30 to 40 days you should take between 150 to 300 billion or more probiotics per day. This will ensure a quick repopulation of good bacteria in your gut.

- **CoQ10** 200 to 400mg once to twice per day with food.

If Constipation, Digestive Problems, Stage 3 or 4 Kidney Disease or You Would Like To Be Very Aggressive In YourCare, You Can Use Acacia Fiber

- **Acacia Fiber (aka Acacia Gum)** 25 to 50 grams per day in two or three divided doses with food or without. Higher doses are preferred.

CHAPTER8 THE CORE NATURAL KIDNEY HEALTH SUPPLEMENTS EXPLAINED & PRODUCT RECOMMENDATIONS

After each supplement explanation, we provide recommended brands and products to use with amounts per day. There are many good quality supplement companies on the market. Many other brands and products can be used in place of the recommendations. We reference Now Foods supplement company often as they are available around the world, have the highest quality manufacturing available and are affordable for the average person.

- **Multivitamin** - People with chronic kidney disease and especially those in advanced stages, such as 3 to 5, have a high rate of vitamin and mineral deficiencies. The high rate of deficiencies is related to decreased intake, impaired production, concurrent illnesses, and diet restrictions. These deficiencies lead to complications and further free radical and inflammation damage to the kidney. It has been shown that supplementation with a good multivitamin corrects this and improves all outcomes.

For kidney disease, a multivitamin should be low in Vitamin A, which has been shown to be elevated in CKD, and have adequate amounts of all other nutrients especially B vitamins, zinc, vitamin C & E.

Multivitamin

Life Extension Foundation

5990 North Federal Highway

Fort Lauderdale, FL 33308

1-800-544-4440

www.lef.org

Product: Two Per Day Multivitamin

Take 1 pill per day, even though the label states two. The reason is that two pills will have you consuming higher doses of certain vitamins that should be limited in CKD. \

- **Fish Oil** – Fish oil supplements have been shown to be very kidney friendly with many benefits for preventing and slowing CKD. Fish oil is an omega-3 fatty acid.

There are two types of omega-3 fatty acids. Short-chain omega-3 fatty acids are ALA (alpha-linolenic acid). These are found in plants such as flaxseed. Though beneficial, ALA omega-3 fatty acids do not provide the large amount of benefits that long-chain omega-3 fatty acids do.

Long-chain omega-3 fatty acids are EPA (eicosapentaenoic acid) and DHA (docosahexaenoic acid). The EPA and DHA are the types that have shown benefit in kidney disease and other complications such as cardiovascular problems.

The EPA and DHA will need to be in a therapeutic dose which will be listed on the label of the fish oil bottle. You will want the **EPA to be 1500mg up to 5000mg and DHA 1000 up to 4000mg.**

Omega-3 Fatty Acids as Fish Oil

Most liquid fish oils have been molecular distilled and free of toxins. Listed below are two good quality, pleasant tasting fish oils. Do not use cod liver oil because of the higher content of vitamin A. **Take 2 teaspoons to 1 tablespoon of liquid fish oil per day. For pills you will need 4 pills per day. 2 pills taken twice per day.** We also offer a unique omega 3 blend for kidney disease called Kidney Shield.

Healthy Kidney Publishing

501 North Avenue Gf

Wood-Ridge, NJ 07075

1-800-927-1738

www.healthykidneyinc.com

Product: Kidney Shield™

Lemon flavor

2 pills twice per day

Carlson Laboratories

15 W College Drive

Arlington Heights, Illinois 60004

1-800-323-4141

www.carlsonlabs.com

Product: The Very Finest Fish Oil

Comes in orange of lemon flavor

2 teaspoons (tsp) to 1 tablespoon (tbsp.) per day

- **Vitamin D3 (Cholecalciferol if needed)** - The "sunshine vitamin," so named because it is synthesized in your skin from sun exposure, has been shown to help every aspect of kidney disease. Vitamin D deficiency is found in about 79% of kidney disease sufferers and higher doses show many benefits.

The two major forms are vitamin D2 or ergocalciferol (synthetic), and vitamin D3 or cholecalciferol (natural). D2 is often given as a prescription and studies show it benefits the kidneys, but the natural form D3 has shown additional benefits over D2.

You will want to consume Vitamin D3 as cholecalciferol and **take**

2000 to 5000IU per day. It is also preferred to take a formula with K2 in it.

Vitamin D3 & K2

NOW Foods

395 S. Glen Ellyn Road

Bloomingdale, IL 60108

1-888-669-3663

www.nowfoods.com

Product: Vitamin D3 & K2

They have 2 types of products, 1 with 2000IUs and 1 with 5000IUs of Vitamin D. Take 1 pill per day of either product.

Monitoring Blood Work For Vitamin D3 (Cholecalciferol)

The most appropriate marker for vitamin D is 25-hydroxy vitamin D. Most laboratory reference ranges will be from 30 to 100 ng/ml. The optimum dose is between 40 to 60 ng/ml.

If you are not sure of your blood level of Vitamin D then **begin by taking 2,000IUs per day.**

- **Sodium Bicarbonate (if needed)** – One of the kidney's jobs is to keep acidity-alkalinity in balance. If too much acidity builds up, it will cause further kidney damage. This problem can easily be fixed with supplementation of oral sodium bicarbonate tablets *aka* "baking soda."

This treatment is known by some nephrologists, but tends to be used when severe stages of acidity are present. Modern day kidney experts recommend beginning treatment with small doses of sodium bicarbonate earlier in the kidney disease process. This takes the stress off the kidneys and can lead to a slowing of kidney disease.

Some physicians believe they should not give sodium bicarbonate because it may result in sodium retention, elevated blood pressure and edema. These fears have been unfounded, as the main side effect listed is edema which can be corrected by a diuretic which would prevent sodium retention. However, if your sodium intake is low this shouldn't be an issue. In fact, sodium bicarbonate is about 28% of actual sodium and the remaining being bicarbonate. This is less sodium than most pieces of bread.

Sodium bicarbonate is sold over the counter and comes in 10 grain tablets, 1 grain equals 650mg. You will most likely find this product online, as it is not commonly carried in most pharmacies. You also can use baking soda, if you can stand the taste.

Begin taking ½ **tablet to1 tablet per day between meals** to avoid belching and bloating. You can also take ½ **to1 teaspoon per day of baking soda**. This amount can be increased or lowered depending on your blood work.

You can also purchase an enteric coated sodium bicarbonate which can be taken anytime. The enteric coating prevents the sodium bicarbonate from releasing in the stomach avoiding any digestive discomfort.

Sodium Bicarbonate

Any sodium bicarbonate tablet is fine to take for short term. Short term being 6-12 months. It should be 10g (650mg) per pill. You will find sodium bicarbonate on amazon.com or by searching it online. It's typically not carried in supplement stores.

It is preferred to use enteric coated sodium bicarbonate tablets for long term. Enteric coated tablets prevent the sodium bicarbonate from releasing in the stomach, thereby preventing adverse effects. Instead, it is released in the small intestine where no adverse effects occur.

Healthy Kidney Publishing

501 North Avenue Gf

Wood-Ridge, NJ 07075

1-800-927-1738

www.healthykidneyinc.com

Product: Kidney Restore™

This is our product with a combination of probiotics and sodium bicarbonate that is enteric coated to support normal kidney function. **Take 2 to 4 pills per day.**

Monitoring Blood Work for the Acid-Alkaline Balance

On a blood test you will see the symbol CO_2 which stands for carbon dioxide. You may also find it listed as carbon dioxide. This laboratory test is to measure the amount of CO_2 in your blood.

In the body, most of the CO_2 is in the form of a substance called bicarbonate. Therefore, the CO_2 blood test is really a measure of your blood bicarbonate level, which reflects the acid-alkaline balance.

Most lab reference ranges are about 21 to 33 mmol/l. Your goal should be 22 mmol/l and above using the least amount of sodium bicarbonate. Once in the 22 mmol/l range or above, you should maintain this dose with the least amount of sodium bicarbonate. You should not raise your dose to increase the CO_2 level.

If you are already above 22 mmol/l, but below 26 mmol/l you can take **½ tablet per day or ½ tsp.per day** of baking soda. If you are at 27 mmol/l or above, you do not need to take any sodium bicarbonate. In some cases, higher amounts of sodium bicarbonate, 2 to 3 tablets for example, can be used to reach adequate blood levels of CO_2 of 22 to 27 mmol/l.

Probiotics - As mentioned earlier, probiotics is the term given to multiple beneficial bacteria located in the intestines, which help remove uremic toxins. Two of these probiotics, lactobacillus acidophilus, and bifidobacteriumlongum, have been specifically studied for their kidney benefit and should be consumed by anyone with kidney disease. Each capsule should contain between 60 billion and 100 billion colony forming units made up from the two mentioned probiotics and a variety of others.

The **recommended dose is to take between 1 to 3 pills perday** depending on the strength of the product and preferably on an empty stomach (between meals/snacks). Between meals has shown better absorption of probiotics, but they can be taken with meals if taking them on an empty stomach is difficult.

Probiotic Loading: For the first 30 to 45 days you should consume 150-200 billion probiotics per day. You can even increase your doses to 200 billion or more per day. This has been shown to lower BUN levels, stabilize creatinine and eGFR quickly. After the 30 to 45 days you can continue with high doses, but should consume at least 60 to 100 billion probiotics per day. High doses are generally not needed after the loading phase and maintenance doses are usually adequate. We recommend using our product Kidney Restore™ with an additional 100 billion per pill probiotic.

Healthy Kidney Publishing

501 North Avenue Gf

Wood-Ridge, NJ 07075

1-800-927-1738

www.healthykidneyinc.com

Product: Kidney Restore™

This is our product with a combination of probiotics, sodium bicarbonate that is delayed release to support normal kidney function. **Take 2 to 4 pills per day.**

NOW Foods

395 S. Glen Ellyn Road

Bloomingdale, IL 60108

1-888-669-3663

www.nowfoods.com

Product: Probiotic-10 100 billion

Take **1 to 3 pills per day during loading phase** of a 100 billion probiotic pill per day. Any 100 billion probiotic per pill will be adequate. For best results use along with Kidney Restore™

- **Coenzyme Q10 (CoQ10)** - This substance is similar to a vitamin and is found in every cell of the body and has high concentrations in the kidney. The human body makes CoQ10, and every cell uses it to produce energy for cell growth and maintenance. It also functions as an antioxidant which protects the kidneys and body from damage caused by harmful substances.

The recommended dose of **CoQ10 is 200 to 600mg per day**. This can be taken in one pill per day with food.

NOW Foods

395 S. Glen Ellyn Road

Bloomingdale, IL 60108

1-888-669-3663

www.nowfoods.com

Product: Any CoQ10 product that is 200mg or more. **Take 1 to 2 pills** per day.

- **Acacia Fiber -** Also known as acacia gum, gum arabic, chaargund, char goond, or meska, and is a natural gum made of hardened sap taken from two species of the acacia tree; acacia senegal and acacia seyal. Acacia fiber has the ability to remove damaging kidney toxins from the body safely.

Acacia fiber is an extremely therapeutic agent that shows benefit at any stage of kidney disease. You can use this at any point in your kidney disease. If you are close to kidney failure, I recommend reading Chapter 9for using acacia fiber to avoid kidney failure and dialysis.

The recommended dose is **25 to 50 grams per daywith food or**

empty stomach in two of three divided doses. Gradually increase the fiber till desired amounts are reached.

NOW Foods

395 S. Glen Ellyn Road

Bloomingdale, IL 60108

1-888-669-3663

www.nowfoods.com

Product: Acacia Fiber

Take 2 to 4 tablespoons or more per day

CHAPTER 9 STAGE 4 & 5 KIDNEY DISEASE AND AVOIDING DIALYSIS

If you're like many people reading this book, you may be in kidney failure and may have been told to start or prepare to start dialysis. With the limited amount of time at your disposal, the tips below have helped many people avoid dialysis. Use the following recommendations.

- Low to very low protein diet with essential amino acids.

- Acacia Fiber has been used in the Middle East and other parts of the world to help people avoid dialysis based on a body weight dosage. Recommendation is to divide your acacia fiber doses into two or three times per day.

- Use probiotics or all supplements from Base Protocol.

- Use any or all supplements listed under your specific condition.

Calculating Acacia Fiber Dosage

Acacia fiber dose should be 1 gram per kilogram of body weight per day.

First, determine your weight in kilograms. Divide your body weight by 2.2 which is 1 kilogram (kg). 1 pound = 2.2 kilograms.

Example: 175 pound person divided by 2.2 gives us the weight in kilograms of 79.

To determine amount of acacia fiber per day, multiply 79 x 1 gram of acacia fiber which gives us a total of 79 grams of acacia fiber per day. This amount should be divided throughout the day in two or three doses. Example, you can take 40mg of acacia fiber twice per day for a total of 80 grams.

If taking these high doses of acacia fiber is not feasible. Take at least 50 grams per day. 50 grams and higher has shown tremendous benefits.

NOW Foods

395 S. Glen Ellyn Road

Bloomingdale, IL 60108

1-888-669-3663

www.nowfoods.com

Product: Acacia Fiber

CHAPTER 10 SPECIFIC SUPPLEMENTS FORDIFFERENT DISEASES

This chapter covers specific supplements for the most common types of kidney disease. Not every issue that can cause kidney disease will be covered here, however, feel free to take advantage of your email support to have the program personalized for your issues and contact us with any questions.

Ideally, you would be taking the core supplements, previously listed, and can add in any additional supplements for more kidney support.

If you don't see your condition listed please contact customer support to speak to one of our healthy kidney coaches. support@healthykidneyinc.com

Diabetes

Diabetic nephropathy (diabetes induced kidney disease) occurs when the blood sugar is not controlled and off balance. Since diabetic nephropathy is caused by unstable blood sugar which damages the kidney, it's best to stabilize the blood sugar to halt kidney damage with a proper diet, and nutritional supplements will help to maintain and improve kidney health

Supplement Guidelines for Diabetic Nephropathy

- **Milk Thistle Extract (Silymarin) Botanical Name: SilybumMarianum** Milk thistle has been used medicinally for more than 2,000 years. A flavonoid complex called silymarin can be extracted from the seeds of milk thistle and is the biologically active component. The terms "milk thistle" and "silymarin" are often used interchangeably. Milk thistle products are popular in Europe and the US for the management of various types of liver disease.

Milk thistle extract has been shown to benefit kidney disease in animal studies and in humans with diabetic nephropathy. The recommended dose is **milk thistle extract standardized to 150 to 300mg per pill two to three times per day with food.**

NOW Foods

395 S. Glen Ellyn Road

Bloomingdale, IL 60108

1-888-669-3663

www.nowfoods.com

Product: Milk Thistle Extract. A variety of milk thistle extract strengths are available. From 150 to 300mg per pill. Best to purchase the higher dose products. **Take 2 to 3 pillsper day**

Alpha Lipoic Acid - This antioxidant is made by the body and is found in every cell, where it helps turn glucose into energy. This powerful substance has shown to protect the kidney, safely excrete heavy metal toxins, control blood sugar in diabetics and improve many CKD symptoms.

The recommended dose is **600mg once to twice per day with food.**

NOW Foods

395 S. Glen Ellyn Road

Bloomingdale, IL 60108

1-888-669-3663

www.nowfoods.com

Product: Alpha Lipoic Acid 600 mg per pill.

Take 1 to 2 pills per day.

- **GymnemaSylvestre** leaves have been used for more than 2,000 years in India to treat diseases.It has shown to control Type 1 and Type 2 diabetes and have some kidney protecting effects.

Take GymnemaSylvestre Extract 200 to 400mgper pill twice per day with food.

NOW Foods

395 S. Glen Ellyn Road

Bloomingdale, IL 60108

1-888-669-3663

www.nowfoods.com

Product: GymnemaSylvestre 400 mg

Take 1 pill twice per day

- **Vitamin B6 (Pyridoxine & P-5-P)**This B vitamin has shown to slow down further progression of kidney disease related to diabetes and can reduce protein in the urine. B6 comes in different forms.

Take B6 as Pyridoxine or P-5-P (Pyridoxal-5-Phosphate) 100mg per day.

Product: Many brands offer Pyridoxine or P-5-P. Pills come in 50 to 100mg. Take 100mg once per day.

Hypertension

Hypertension (high blood pressure) must be controlled in CKD. It can be a cause of kidney disease or develop from a loss of kidney function. If the kidney loses too much function the hormones it produces to control blood pressure become imbalanced. This imbalance leads to high blood pressure and further loss of kidney function.

Hypertension induced kidney disease can be helped with:

- CoQ10 & Omega-3 – Take 200mg of CoQ10 twice per day. Also use higher dose omega-3s. You will want the EPA to be around 2400mg up and DHA 1000mg or more up once per day.

Monitoring Hypertension

Those with kidney disease should monitor their blood pressure, especially when starting new diet and lifestyle changes. There are two ways to monitor your blood pressure: either with an electronic device, or a manual one with a stethoscope and blood pressure cuff.

The electronic devices can be unreliable, so it is best to learn how to take your own blood pressure with an inexpensive stethoscope. It will take a bit of practice, but it has shown to be the most reliable method. The reasons are is it gives you an average of many readings and eliminates anxiety-producing doctor visits. If you do decide to use an electronic device take multiple readings, on both arms and calculate your average blood pressure.

Nutritional & Herbal Supplements, Medications and Hypertension

There are many nutritional and herbal supplements that can lower blood pressure. However, it is better to take prescription medications and here is why.

The effective natural and herbal supplements, like certain doses and forms of potassium, can build up levels in CKD causing complications. No one with CKD should be taking potassium supplements.

Herbal supplements shown effective for blood pressure have not been studied in CKD thoroughly, so they should be avoided. We don't know what the side effects are or what complications may arise.

Medications for blood pressure are very effective and the best route to pursue. Certain classes, such as Angiotensin-Converting Enzyme (ACE) Inhibitors and Angiotensin II Receptor Blockers (ARB), have shown to control blood pressure and slow down kidney disease. This is why working with a knowledgeable medical doctor is a must, so they can prescribe the best conventional or allopathic medicines in conjunction with the The Complete Guide to Supplements for Kidney Health   Kidney Health Program.

Polycystic Kidney Disease and other Cystic Diseases

Polycystic kidney disease (PKD) and other cystic diseases arecharacterized by clusters of cysts developingwithin the kidneys causing them to enlarge and lose function. The more cysts there are or the larger the size of the cysts, the greater damage is done to the kidneys.

Supplement and dietary recommendations that have shown to benefit cystic diseases and PKD:

- **Consume soy proteins** in the form of non gmo tofu, tempuh, and edamame beans 3 to 4 times per week.

- **2 tablespoons of flax seeds** per day. Whole or grinded flaxseeds can be used and slow cyst growth.

- **Consume at least half** your body weight in ounces of water per day. Proper hydration has shown to be very important in cystic diseases. Proper hydrations lowers vasopressin, a hormone, where lower levels slow down cyst development.

- **Sodium Bicarbonate** – Even if metabolic acidosis is not present, a daily dose has shown to prevent cyst formation in PKD. Sodium bicarbonate can also be used in other cystic diseases.

Take **325 to 650mg of sodium bicarbonate** once per day.

Healthy Kidney Publishing

501 North Avenue Gf

Wood-Ridge, NJ 07075

1-800-927-1738

www.healthykidneyinc.com

Product: Kidney Restore™

This is our product with a combination of probiotics, sodium bicarbonate that is enteric coated to support normal kidney function. **Take 1 to 2 pills per day.**

There are many other sodium bicarbonate pills on the market that can be used in place of Kidney Restore™.

- **Curcumin** – Known as Turmeric extract benefits nearly every organ system including the kidneys. Curcumin inhibits inflammatory factors, supports immune system function, promotes heart health, and offers potent antioxidant protection. Curcumin is difficult to absorb, so a certain curcumin formula that has BCM-95® Bio-Curcumin® extract is preferred for the kidneys.

Life Extension Foundation

5990 North Federal Highway

Fort Lauderdale, FL 33308

1-800-544-4440

www.lef.org

Product: Super Bio-Curcumin®

A highly absorbable curcumin product. Take 3 pills per day in two of three divided doses with food.

- **Resveratrol** - Is a plant nutrient with several therapeutic effects. It has been shown to exert anti-inflammatory and anti-oxidative effects, and affect the progression and initial of many diseases.

NOW Foods

395 S. Glen Ellyn Road

Bloomingdale, IL 60108

1-888-669-3663

www.nowfoods.com

Product: Natural Resveratrol 200 mg Veg Capsules

Take 2 to 4 pills per day in two of three divided doses.

Conjugated Linoleic Acid (CLA)− CLA is a naturally occurring fatty acid found in meat and dairy products that has shown benefits for PKD.

Product: Any company that offers 1000mg per pill. Take 2 pills twice per day.

Malformations (congenital anomalies of the kidney)

Malformations that occur as a baby develops in its mother's womb. For example, a narrowing may occur that prevents normal outflow of urine and causes urine to flow back up to the kidney. This causes infections and may damage the kidneys.

The amount of congenital anomalies of the kidneys is extremely broad and ranges from mild, no symptom malformations such as a double ureter to life-threatening issues like bilateral renal agenesis.

- For malformations follow the base supplement protocol and use recommendations for specific issues that may arise.

IgA nephropathy also known as Berger's disease

IgA nephropathy, also known as Berger's disease, is a kidney disease that occurs when an antibody called immunoglobulin A (IgA) becomes lodged in the kidneys resulting in inflammation that, over time, may hamper your kidneys' ability to filter wastes from your blood.

No cure exists for IgA nephropathy, but keeping blood pressure and cholesterol under control and the using this program can slow or stop progression of the disease.

- **Omega-3** – In IgA nephropathy maximizing your omega-3 intake is crucial. Make sure to use the upper limits of intake as discussed in its section. Use 1 tbsp of liquid fish oil or 4 to as much as 6 omega-3 pills per day.

- **Tripterygium Wilfordii Hook F (aka. Thunder god root, thunder god, thunder god vine or lei gong teng) -**

Thunder god vine is a perennial grown in Taiwan and China. It has been used for hundreds of years in traditional Chinese medicine to treat swelling caused by inflammation.

Currently, thunder god vine is used as a dietary supplement for autoimmune diseases and has shown tremendous benefits for IgA nephropathy. A meta-analysis (grouping of studies of 188 people) has shown that thundergod root can lower proteinuria, reduce inflammation and many cases went into remission.

Thunder God Root

PO Box 1154

Pataskala, OH 43062

Phone: 903-883-7668

www.thundergodrootextract.com

Product: Thunder God Vine Root 20:1 Capsules 200mg 90 Count. Take 1 pill per day with food.

Artemisia Absinthium which is commonly called absinthe or wormwood, is a woody-based perennial that is grown for its attractive silver-gray foliage that has many therapeutic benefits. In IgA nephropathy it has showed a significant reduction in proteinuria and arterial blood pressure in the early stages of IgA.

Allergy Research Group LLC

2300 North Loop Road

Alameda, CA 94502

Phone: 1-800-545-9960

Product: Artemisia 100 Vegetarian Capsules

Take 3 pills per day in two to three divided doses.

- **Gluten Free Diet** - IgA is a major antibody of the gastrointestinal tract, and a study showed that 75% of patients had an improvement in proteinuria with a gluten-free diet. One-third of patients with IgA nephropathy demonstrate sensitivity to gluten. A gluten-free diet must be started early in the disease process. Many patients showed improvement but continued to progress toward kidney failure.

A gluten free diet can be used as part of a program to help your kidneys. A gluten-free diet is a diet that excludes the protein gluten. Gluten is found in grains. You will need to read ingredient labels to avoid all sources of gluten. Gluten is in wheat (including wheat varieties like spelt, kamut, farro and durum, plus products like bulgar and semolina), barley, rye, triticale and oats

- **Aspirin** –Case reports have shown that when omega-3 high in EPA was used in conjunction with low dose aspirin rates of remission were much higher.

Aspirin is controversial when it comes to kidney disease. For the most part it is avoided when CKD is present. However, the research is inconclusive when recommending for all kidney diseases. However, the benefits shown in IgA are excellent. Discuss with your doctor before taking.

Product: Any safety coated baby aspirin that is 81mg. Many brands available such as Bayer.

Glomerulonephritis

Glomerulonephritis, AKA glomerular nephritis, is something of a catch-all term referring to several different diseases which usually affect both kidneys. These diseases are typically characterized by inflammation of the small blood vessels in the kidneys known as glomeruli. Glomerulonephritis can be caused due to a problem with the body's immune system or from taking certain medications (like NSAIDs) or even as result of certain kinds of streptococcal infections.

As it is not strictly a single disease, its presentation depends on the specific disease entity: it may present with isolated hematuria and/or proteinuria (blood or protein in the urine); or as a nephrotic (primarily marked by protein loss) syndrome, a nephritic (primarily marked by blood loss) syndrome, acute kidney injury, or chronic kidney disease.

It can be further categorized into:

Focal Segmental Glomerulosclerosis

Focal segmental glomerulosclerosis (FSGS) is a disease in which scar tissue develops on the glomeruli. It is a serious condition that can lead to kidney failure. Treatment options for FSGS depend on the type you have.

Types of FSGS include:

- **Primary FSGS.** Some people diagnosed with FSGS have no known cause for their condition. This is referred to as primary or idiopathic FSGS.

- **Secondary FSGS.** This is the term reserved for FSGS caused by a variety of different potential factors, ranging from infections to drug toxicity or even diseases such as diabetes, obesity, sickle cell disease or other forms of kidney disease. Treating or managing the underlying cause can oftenstopresulting kidney damage and may even help improve kidney function.

- **Genetic (also called familial) FSGS.** This is the rarest type of FSGS; it istypically caused by a genetic mutation. It's more likely to occur in families with an established history of the disease, however, familial FSGS can also occur in instances where neither parent has the disease if each parent has one copy of the abnormal gene responsible for FSGS and passes it on to their children.

Recommendations For FSGS

- **Reishi (Ganoderma lucidum),** commonly known as Ling

Zhi in Chinese, is a herbal mushroom that is useful to treat FSGS. In a small studyall individuals achieved remission by a reduction of inflammation.

Life Extension Foundation

5990 North Federal Highway

Fort Lauderdale, FL 33308

1-800-544-4440

www.lef.org

Product: Reishi Extract Mushroom Complex - 60 Vegetarian Capsules Take 1 capsule twice per day with meals.

- **Vitamin E**is a fat-soluble nutrient found in many foods. In the body and in the kidneys, it acts as an antioxidant, helping to protect cells from the damage caused by free radicals. It has shown benefits in FSGS.

NOW Foods

395 S. Glen Ellyn Road

Bloomingdale, IL 60108

1-888-669-3663

www.nowfoods.com

Product: Vitamin E-400 Mixed Tocopherols - 100 Softgels. Take

1 pill per day.

- **CoQ10** as discussed earlier is a potent supplement for kidney disease. It has shown excellent benefits in FSGS, and therefore should be increased to 400-600mg per day in two of three doses.

- **Vitamin A** is another fat-soluble nutrient found in many foods and acts as an antioxidant. It has shown benefits in FSGS.

NOW Foods

395 S. Glen Ellyn Road

Bloomingdale, IL 60108

1-888-669-3663

www.nowfoods.com

Product: Vitamin A 25,000IU per pill. Take 1 pill per day for 60-90 days and discontinue.

- **Membranous Glomerulonephritisn** Membranous glomerulonephritisis typified by the glomerulibecoming damaged and thickened. As a result, proteins leak from the glomeruli and find their way into the urine leading to proteinuria. For many, loss of these proteins eventually causes signs and symptoms known as nephrotic syndrome.

The listed supplements have shown antioxidant benefits and astragalus has case reports of remission in membranous glomerulonephritis.

- **Astragalus (Astragalus membranaceous)** This herb comes from the root of a perennial plant that grows in the northern and eastern parts of China as well as in Korea. Astragalus has shown tremendous benefits in membranous glomerulonephritis.

Puritans Pride LLC

4320 Veterans Memorial Hwy

Holbrook, NY 11741

1- 800 645-1030

https://www.puritan.com

Product: Astragalus Extract 1000 mgper pill. Take 5 pills three times per day. For a total of 15 pills. This may seem like a lot of pills, however that was used in the studies and shown to help reach remission.

The following three supplements N-A-C, Vitamin C and Vitamin E should be used all together. The reason being that the study used all the nutrients combined for high antioxidant benefits in membranous glomerulonephritis.

- **N-Acetyl-Cysteine (a.k.a. "N-A-C")** N-Acetyl-Cysteine

comes from the amino acid L-cysteine and restores the body glutathione level. Glutathione is one of the body's most abundant anti-oxidants, and has shown to be low in kidney disease and is restored with supplementation which can protect the kidneys. The recommended dose is 600-1000mg twice per day.

NOW Foods

395 S. Glen Ellyn Road

Bloomingdale, IL 60108

1-888-669-3663

www.nowfoods.com

Product: NOW Foods NAC 1000 mg per pill. Take 1 pill twice per day.

- **Vitamin C** also known as L-ascorbic acid, is a water-soluble vitamin that is naturally found in some foods, and available as a dietary supplement. It has potent anti-oxidant benefits. There are a variety of forms of vitamin c. I recommend using the Ester-C form of vitamin c. It has a better absorption rate and non-acidic.

American Health Sciences

2100 Smithtown Avenue

Ronkonkoma NY 11779

1-800-445-7137

Product: Ester-C purchase 500 or 1000mg with Citrus Bioflavonoids per capsule. Take 1000 to 1500mg per day in one to two divided doses.

- **Vitamin E** has tremendous antioxidant benefits formembranous glomerulonephritis, helping to protect cells from the damage caused by free radicals.

NOW Foods

395 S. Glen Ellyn Road

Bloomingdale, IL 60108

1-888-669-3663

www.nowfoods.com

Product: Vitamin E-400 Mixed Tocopherols - 100 Softgels. Take 1 pill twice per day.

Mesangial Proliferative Glomerulonephritis

Mesangial Proliferative Glomerulonephritis (MPGN) is characterized by an increased number of mesangial cells in the glomeruli in the kidneys which cause damage to the glomeruli. It's been known to be present alongside nephrotic syndrome, which typically includes symptoms such as proteinuria, low blood protein levels, high cholesterol levels, high triglyceride levels, and swelling. Blood in the urine is sometimes also a symptom.

- **Alpha Lipoic Acid** -This antioxidant discussed early has shown benefits for MPGN. It can help reduce the free radicals found in high amounts in MPGN.

The recommended dose is 600mg once to twice per day with food.

NOW Foods

395 S. Glen Ellyn Road

Bloomingdale, IL 60108

1-888-669-3663

www.nowfoods.com

- **Rosmarinic Acid** - Rosmarinic acid is a plant-based compound found in a wide variety of spices. Most well known for being the active ingredient in Rosemary. It has anti-inflammatory and anti-oxidant effects, and may slow the progression of MPGN.

Swanson Health Products

www.swansonvitamins.com

P.O. Box 2803

Fargo, ND 58108-2803

1-800-451-9304

Product: Swanson Superior HerbsRosemary Extract. Take 2 pills three times per day.

- **Rhurbarb (Rheum)** - Rhubarb has shown beneficial for MPGN. Rhubarb is a vegetable with a unique taste that makes it a favorite in manypies and desserts. It grows in the wild in the mountains of the Western and Northwestern provinces of China and in the adjoining Tibetan territory, and is cultivated in much of Europe and the US.

The recommended dose of rhubarb is 4,000 to 9,000mg per day in two or (evenbetter) three divided doses with food. Example: 2,000mg twice per day,3,000mg three times per day or 4,000mg twice per day, etc.

Warning: Rhubarb has a high oxalic content and must be avoided by anyone with ahistory or at risk for kidney stones. Also, avoid if you have atherosclerosis.

Nature's Answer

1-800-439-2324

www.naturesanswer.com

Product: Rhubarb Root. Each dropper full is 2,000mg. Take 1 to 4 droppers per day in two or threedivided doses.

Lupus Nephritis

Lupus is an autoimmune disease stemming from the immune system attacking its own tissues and organs. Lupus-associated inflammation often targets multiple organs at once, but can be particularly devastating to the kidneys. This form of kidney disease is called lupus nephritis.

- **Omega-3** – Maximize your omega-3 . Make sure to use the upper limits of intake as discussed in its section. Use 1 tbsp of liquid fish oil or 4 to as much as 6 omega-3 pills per day.

- **Cordyceps Sinensis**has been described as a medicine in old Chinese medical books and Tibetan medicine. It is a rare combination of a fungus that grows on a caterpillar, and a species of cordyceps is used to make an anti-rejection medication.

NOW Foods

395 S. Glen Ellyn Road

Bloomingdale, IL 60108

1-888-669-3663

www.nowfoods.com

Product: Cordyceps 750 mg Vegetarian Capsules

Take 2 pills twice per day

- **Artemisia Absinthium** which is commonly called absinthe or wormwood, is a woody-based perennial that is grown for its attractive silver-gray foliage that has many therapeutic benefits. In IgA nephropathy it has showed a significant reduction in proteinuria and arterial blood pressure in the early stages of IgA.

Allergy Research Group LLC

2300 North Loop Road

Alameda, CA 94502

Phone: 1-800-545-9960

Product: Artemisia 100 Vegetarian Capsules

Take 3 pills per day in two to three divided doses

Nephritis

Nephritis occurs when your kidneys suddenly become inflamed. This could be for a variety of reasons, however, if left untreated it could lead to kidney failure. Various types of nephritis are covered in their appropriate sections, ie: Lupus Nephritis, we are covering interstitial and pyelonephritis below.

There are a few types of acute nephritis:

- **Interstitial nephritis** This form of nephritis is marked by the spaces between the kidney tubules becoming inflamed, which in turn, causes the kidneys to swell.

- **Pyelonephritis** This kind of nephritis is usually due to a bacterial infection, especially repeated urinary tract infections. It typically originates in the bladder, making its way through the ureters and then to the kidneys.

Recommendations

- **Followappropriate** diet, use base supplement protocol and can add in any supplements from, "Additional Supplement" chapter and Acute Kidney Injury Section below.

Kidney Transplant

Kidney transplant or renal transplant is an organ transplant of a kidney into a person with kidney failure. Kidney transplants are from living-donor transplants depending on the source of the organ donor or deceased-donors (known as a cadaver kidney).

The main reason for me entering the field of holistic health and focusing on kidney disease is, because my own kidney transplant. I refused to accept the fate of a donor kidney lasting for a period of time and needing to go through kidney failure, dialysis and a kidney transplant again. I have used these same recommendations myself.

- **Follow appropriate diet**, use base supplement protocol and can add in any antioxidant supplements from,

"Additional Supplements" chapter and if you have problems with organ rejection. The herb cordyceps has shown benefit and safety with transplant medications. I highly recommend contacting us for email support to personalize the program to your kidney transplant situation.

Our Complete Guide to Renal Diet Plans &Cookbooks is also an invaluable resource for identifying which of the three best kidney diets (low protein, vegetarian or Academy of Dieticians) would be ideal for you.

Obstructions

Obstructions caused by problems like kidney stones, tumors or an enlarged prostate gland in men. Treat the obstructive causes with conventional medicine.

- **Follow appropriate diet**, use base supplement protocol and can add in any supplements from, "Additional Supplements" chapter.

Recommendations For Kidney Stones

Kidney Stonesalso called(nephrolithiasis or renal lithiasis,) are hard deposits made of salts and minerals that form inside your kidneys.

- **Follow appropriate diet** with additional dietary recommendations listed. All the dietary recommendations have shown to reduce the risk of kidney stones. ½ ounce of rice, oat, or wheat bran added to your diet daily. One study found that drinking 2 liters of lemonade per day helped prevent kidney stones. Avoid coffee and tea. Coffee and tea increase urinary oxalate excretion, possibly increasing risk of stones. Limit your intake of spinach, rhubarb, beet greens, nuts, chocolate, almonds, peanuts, and strawberries, which appear to significantly increase urinary oxalate levels. Consume a handful of pumpkin seeds daily which reduces the risk of kidney stone formation.

- **Magnesium Citrate** has shown to reduce stone formation in doses of 500-600mg per day.

NOW Foods

395 S. Glen Ellyn Road

Bloomingdale, IL 60108

1-888-669-3663

www.nowfoods.com

Product: Now Foods Magnesium Citrate 200mg, 250 Tablets. Take 3 pills per day in two of three divided doses. There are many available brands of magnesium citrate available on the market.

Acute Kidney Injury

Acute kidney injury refers to a typically rapid loss of kidney function that occurs suddenly, typically in less than a few days. With the kidneys' impaired function, toxins accumulate and your blood's chemical makeup becomes imbalanced. It's most common in people who are already hospitalized or suffering from some other illness.

- **Ginger (Zingiberofficinale)**a very popular ingredient used in cooking, especially in Asian and Indian cuisine. It has been used for medicinal purposes for thousands of years. It has shown to help acute kidney injury from a variety of insults. Such as medications, and environmental toxins.

Pure Encapsulations

490 Boston Post Road

Sudbury, MA 01776 USA

1-800-753-2277

https://www.pureencapsulations.com/

Product: Ginger Extract 500mg per pill.

Take 2 pills twice per day.

- **Nigella Sativa**is an annual flowering plant, native to south and southwest Asia. Its seeds are known by difference names such as black cumin, black caraway, nigella, fennel flower, roman coriander and nutmeg. Supplement forms are taken from oils from the plant. Similar to ginger it has also shown to help acute kidney injury from medications, environmental toxins and diseases.

Life Extension Foundation

5990 North Federal Highway

Fort Lauderdale, FL 33308

1-800-544-4440

www.lef.org

Product: Black Cumin Seed Oil

Take 4 to 6 pills per day in divided doses. Ex: 2 pills twice per day, 3 pills twice per day, 2 pills three times per day.

CHAPTER 11 PROTEIN ENERGY MALNUTRITION (PEM)

Protein–energy malnutrition (PEM) is a form of malnutrition, that is defined as a range of pathological conditions arising from lack of dietary protein. It is secondary to kidney disease. The condition has mild, moderate, and severe degrees. In kidney disease, it's generally not the lack of protein in the diet, it's due to the fact the protein is being lost through the urine.

This is when your doctors tell you to eat more protein. However, more protein will make kidney disease worse. If PEM is present, you are most likely losing lots of protein through your urine.

Therefore, adding more protein to your diet increases metabolic waste that your kidneys have to work harder to remove. Leading to a faster decline in kidney function. The medical doctor's viewpoint is that it's better to have kidney failure with adequate protein levels as opposed to constant PEM, which increases the risk of dying. It's better to be on dialysis than dead is the viewpoint.

It's very sad, but in the United States and many places in the world medical professionals are simply not taught how to correct this issue safely and effectively. This is not a new treatment just one that has only recently begun being published in current medical books. It has been used for decades obscurely in the US, but has become a standard of care in some countries.

To understand this condition, and how to correct it we must first understand protein and amino acids.

Protein

Protein is a macronutrient that is essential to building muscle mass and is needed for every biological process in the body. Without adequate protein you cannot live. Protein is made up of amino acids. Your body digests the protein you eat into individual amino acids and uses those amino acids for every process in the body.

When the correct amino acids are taken orally, they provide your body with the protein it needs without any metabolic waste. Therefore, improving PEM and helping a variety of kidney diseases.

Essential Amino Acids & Amino Acids

There are 20 amino acids and 12 are considered non-essential because the body can manufacture them. The other 8 need to be consumed from supplemental sources in order to keep an adequate nutritional balance.

One amino acid called L-Histidine is considered a semi-essential amino acid because adults generally produce adequate amounts, but children may not. However, in kidney disease it is believed the body lacks the ability to produce histidine, therefore it will need to be consumed along with the 8 essential amino acids.

The 8 essential amino acids are:

- Isoleucine

- L-Leucine

- L-Lysine

- L-Methionine

- L-Phenylalanine

- L-Threonine

- L-Tryptophan

- L-Valine

You will need to consume anywhere from 3.0 to 4.0 grams of essential amino acids and histidine once to three times per day with meals. With most commercial essential amino acid products available, this will come out to 4 to 7 pills once to three times per day with meals. The mixture of amino acids can also be taken as a powder.

In many cases, you can consume fewer pills and powders depending on your protein consumption and albumin blood work numbers, which is discussed on the following pages.

Here is a list of each milligram dose of essential amino acids and l-histidine required at one to three times per day to avoid protein malnutrition. If you use a product and are close to the following numbers, that is usually sufficient to help your situation. I have also seen many people improve PED without histidine. It is preferable to take of course, but with the amount of changes people will have to make, this can sometimes feel overwhelming.

Therefore, *any* of the products recommended are beneficial and provide what is needed.

- L-Isoleucine, 400mg

- L-Leucine, 600mg

- L-Lysine, 400mg

- L-Methionine, 600mg

- L-Phenylalanine, 600mg

- L-Threonine, 300mg

- L-Tryptophan, 150mg

- L-Valine, 500mg

- L-Histidine, 300mg

There have also been many people who have purchased essential amino acids individually and in combined quantities and have been able to make up the recommended amounts.

For example, you can use an L-lysine pill that is 500mg per day three times per day to meet your daily protein nutritional need of that amino acid. You can also use BCAA (Branch Chained Amino Acids) pills or powders which are made up of L-Leucine, L-Isoleucine, and L-Valine to meet amino acid nutritional needs.

There are also mixtures of the essential amino acids, in smaller doses, along with other non-essential amino acids in pill and powder forms readily available. This can be combined with essential amino acids to prevent protein malnutrition, but since smaller doses are used, you will need to consume larger amounts of pills and powders.

Depending on your access to essential amino acids, there can be many options available to prevent protein malnutrition and help your kidneys. Ideally, you should strive to use only the essential amino acids and not the non-essential amino acids as this approach has shown the most benefit in kidney disease.

Monitoring Blood Work for Protein Malnutrition

There is a blood test called albumin which is the major protein in blood; albumin (the same name as the test) plays an important role in maintaining fluid balance (osmotic pressure) inside blood vessels, in transporting drugs, hormones, and enzymes, and is further used to determine protein malnutrition.

When low albumin levels are seen in kidney disease, albumin is leaking from the blood into the urine and being lost. This is known as proteinuria.

This blood test range is from 3.5 to 5.5 g/dl. For optimal status you will want to keep your albumin 4.0 g/dl or higher. Dropping under 4.0 g/dl is considered protein deficiency and poorer outcomes in CKD are seen. If you are below 4.0 g/dl an increase in essential amino acids is needed. If your blood test albumin count is 4.5 g/dl or greater you can consume fewer essential amino acid supplements, but you don't have to. Being above 4.0 g/dl is completely fine. However, if you find consuming the supplements difficult and you are above 4.5 g/dl you can reduce the amounts, but make sure to be 4.0 g/dl or greater.

CHAPTER 12 ESSENTIAL AMINO ACID PRODUCTS

Where To Purchase Essential Amino Acid Supplements

You can contact Healthy Kidney Inc. for any supplement purchases you require. Additionally, the websites listed below often carry the aforementioned products.

http://healthykidneyinc.com/
http://nowfoods.com/

http://www.amazon.com/

http://www.vitacost.com/

http://www.camformulas.com/

http://www.rockwellnutrition.com/

http://www.luckyvitamin.com/

http://www.iherb.com/

Companies and Products

Essential Amino Acids

Healthy Kidney Inc.

501 North Avenue, Ground Floor

Wood-Ridge, NJ 07075

1-800-927-1738

http://healthykidneyinc.com/

Product: Pure Kidney Amino Acid Tablets. Our product is exactly formulated for kidney health. Other essential amino acid products are not in ratios designed for kidney health. However, they can be used. Take 5 tablets once to twice daily or as directed by physician.

NOW Foods

395 S. Glen Ellyn Road

Bloomingdale, IL 60108

1-888-669-3663

http://www.nowfoods.com/

Product: Amino-9 Essential Powder

1 ¾ to 2 teaspoons one to three times per day.

Pure Encapsulations

490 Boston Post Road

Sudbury, MA 01776

1-800-753-2277

www.pureencapsulations.com

Product: Essential Amino Acids

Take 6 pills once to twice per day.

Ketoanalogues of Essential Amino Acids Companies

Ketoanalogues of essential amino acids are a combination of essential amino acids and their precursors called ketoanalogues. Ketoanalogue products are 4 to 6 times the cost of essential amino acid products.

However, they are considered 15-25% superior to just using an essential amino acid product by itself. Contact each company for more information about their ketoanalogue products.

Ketorena

1-844-980-9933

sales@nephcentric.com

http://www.ketorena.com

Kidneyhood.org/Albutrix

8383 Greenway Blvd.

Middleton, WI 53562

Tel: 1-800-441-1045

https://www.albutrix.com/

info@kidneyhood.org

CHAPTER 13 CALCIUM, PHOSPHORUS ANDMINERAL BONE DISORDERS

Imbalances of calcium and phosphorus levels in the blood and especially in the bones can be problematic. When phosphorus levels are off, weak and brittle bones can occur, there is poor cell signaling, functioning and energy transfer. This happens because healthy kidneys will maintain these two minerals by converting vitamin D into a more active form called calcitriol. Calcitriol responds to the signals of the parathyroid hormone (PTH) and fibroblast growth factor (FGF-23) to regulate calcium and phosphorus.

Phosphorus

Levels of phosphorus can become imbalanced and thus elevated in stages 3 to 5 when the kidneys start to malfunction. This elevation in phosphorus greatly raises the risk for cardiovascular problems and a higher risk of death.

Phosphorus levels should be checked regularly, and your medical doctor may want to prescribe medication (to be taken with foods) which will decrease the absorption of phosphorus from those foods. High amounts of phosphorus are typically found in large quantities of high protein foods. By following any one of the diets, you will be consuming low amounts of phosphorus which will help to control this level.

If you have high phosphorus levels

The supplement B3 known as niacin and its various forms, such as niacinamide, have been shown to block phosphorus absorption in the digestive track in kidney disease. Thereby naturally lowering the phosphorus level over time. Plus, it helps cholesterol levels and mood.

Niacin has a harmless, but uncomfortable side effect of flushing. A hot and itchy sensation throughout the body. Its harmless and as you take niacin regularly it goes away. To avoid this completely the alternative is to take niacinamide, which has shown to be effective.

B3 (Niacinamide) Take 500-750mg with each meal. Any quality brand can be used such as Now Foods, etc.

Calcium

Levels of calcium are maintained till stages 4 and 5 are reached in CKD. When stages 4 to 5 are present, your doctor may recommend taking a calcium supplement. The blood test for calcium is a poor reflection of how much calcium is in the body, as 1% of the body's calcium is circulating in the blood. Urinary tests have been shown to be more reliable, but this has not become standard medical practice.

The bones cannot properly absorb calcium at these latter stages of kidney disease which leads to weak and brittle bones, easy to fracture. Many doctors will recommend taking calcium supplements in the range of 500 to 1500mg per day to provide more circulating calcium for the bones to absorb. While this excess calcium from supplements and the diet can help the bones, it has led to the concept of "calcium loading." Some of this excess calcium will deposit in other places in the body, including the blood vessels which leads to calcification of arteries and cardiovascular diseases. Calcium absorption will be increased with adequate vitamin d intake, and thus decreasing calcium loading, which is one of the many reasons this nutrient is important to supplement.

Allow your doctor to recommend when and how much calcium in supplemental form to take. Regulating calcium will help with complications of kidney disease, but won't slow or stop the progression of CKD. If you doctor recommends taking calcium supplements, it's also wise to take Vitamin K2. Vitamin K has different forms and K1 is necessary for normal blood clotting and most doctors and health care professionals will be familiar with its various forms and functions. Vitamin K1 (phytonadione) is the natural form of the vitamin which is found in plants, the primary source of the vitamin is through the foods we eat.

Beyond its role in blood clotting, recent research has revealed that vitamin K, specifically K2 (menaquinone), also plays a vital role in maintaining healthy bones and arteries by keeping calcium in the bones and out of the arteries. If you're taking calcium supplements, you can take **K2 in the dose of 30 to 80mcg, or higher, once per day.** This dose may prevent calcium from building up in the arteries.

CHAPTER 14 MANAGING ANEMIA AND FATIGUE

The kidneys play a very important role in preventing anemia, or low red blood cell count, which is a reduction in hemoglobin (Hgb) or hematocrit (Hct) levels. Anemia reduces oxygen-carrying capacity which reduces tissue concentrations and thus fatigue. It also accelerates kidney and cardiovascular diseases, and decreases cognitive functions and overall quality of life.

Anemia in CKD is mostly caused by an inadequate production of erythropoietin, the hormone produced by the kidneys. However, be sure you don't have Protein Energy Malnutrition as discussed in Chapter 18, which can cause fatigue.

According to the World Health Organization, anemia is present when hemoglobin levels fall below 13.0 g/dl. As kidney disease progresses, anemia is very probable, with 90% of those with CKD eventually showing dangerous low levels of red blood cells.

It is commonplace and very beneficial to treat anemia early in the course of CKD. However, this proactive thinking has only shown up in recent years; a good portion of doctors are still going by old standards.

There is a class of medications called Erythropoiesis Stimulating Agents (ESAs), also referred to as epoetin, which are used to raise the Hgb level. Also, in the last 5 years there are additional medications that have come onto the market to improve anemia in CKD. These have been shown to be highly effective, but require a prescription.

The Hemoglobin level on your blood work should be in the range of 11 to 13 g/dl. Keeping the Hemoglobin level between 11 to 12 g/dl has been shown to provide the best benefits. Using medications to raise the level to 13 g/dl or higher has shown negative effects, therefore it should not be your goal.

One troubling fact about medications is that patients need to review their medical insurance coverage plan, as many companies will not provide coverage for these medications unless the (Hgb) hemoglobin drops below 10. Your doctor can still prescribe them, but you will be responsible for a hefty pharmacy bill.

Iron, L-Carnitine, Vitamin C, B12, Folic Acid and Anemia

There are other nutrients (and deficiencies thereof) that can cause, contribute to or help manage anemia in CKD, and improve the effect of ESAs. These nutrients are Iron, L-Carnitine, Vitamin C, B12, and Folic Acid.

- **Iron:** Adequate iron stores are essential both for the body's erythropoietin production and for medications to work.

That's why it is recommended to take a multivitamin with iron.

Your doctor will evaluate your iron levels and advise whether iron supplements are necessary. Constipation, a common side effect of iron supplements, can be corrected by taking a certain form of iron called Iron Bis-Glycinate, *aka* "Gentle Iron." It is highly absorbable and doesn't cause constipation.

- **L-Carnitine:** This carrier molecule helps the body use fats for energy, helps improve anemia, and clear out a toxin called acyl CoA that builds up in kidney disease. Blood tests should be checking for this deficiency when CKD is present.

Correction of the deficiency will not only ease depression, but provide more energy, and improve cognitive function, and quality of life. If you are deficient, you can begin taking **500 to 1500mg per day** and increase your dose based on blood work results.

- **Vitamin C** – This water-soluble vitamin has demonstrated the ability to increase iron absorption. With a good quality multivitamin you will have sufficient intake of vitamin C.

B12 & Folic Acid – Low or deficient numbers of these two B-vitamins will contribute to anemia. The amounts in a multivitamin should be sufficient, however, if your blood work shows you need higher amounts, these B-vitamins can be taken in a separate, higher dose.

CHAPTER 15 MANAGING POTASSIUM PROBLEMS

As mentioned in Chapter 4, in CKD there are two problems with potassium. The most common is having high levels of it, which leads to irregular heartbeats, possible heart attack and possible kidney damage.

High potassium levels are usually seen in stage 3, and more commonly in stages 4 and 5 of CKD. It is often caused by medications and therefore your medical doctor should be making changes accordingly. Your doctor can also prescribe medication to lower the potassium level.

Natural options to control mild to moderately high potassium include using sodium bicarbonate and consuming lower potassium foods. You will most likely have to limit some high potassium fruits and vegetables.

Sodium Bicarbonate ½ tablet (325mg) to 1 tablet (650mg) per day between meals/empty stomach to start.

For dietary recommendations see our book called, "The Complete Guide To Renal Diet Plans & Cook Books" available on Amazon.

CHAPTER 16 MANAGING LOW MAGNESIUM LEVELS

Magnesium, in terms of potential benefits and detriments, continues to attract growing attention in research related to kidney disease. In CKD patients, vascular calcification, hypertension, diabetes, and diabetic nephropathy are common comorbid situations associated with increased risk of death. All of these factors are potentially affected by magnesium, and there is increasing evidence of the beneficial effects of magnesium supplementation and slightly elevated magnesium levels.

In some people with kidney disease or a kidney transplant, there may be low magnesium levels. You can look at your blood work and search for Magnesium, Mag or Mg. If you have a low level you should take a high absorption magnesium supplement. Do not use magnesium oxide. This form will not benefit you. If your magnesium level is close to low, it is up to your discretion whether you should supplement or not.

Pure Encapsulations

490 Boston Post Road

Sudbury, MA 01776

1-800-753-2277

www.pureencapsulations.com

Product: Magnesium Glycinate 120mg per capsule.

Take 1 to 2 pills twice per day.

CHAPTER 17 ADDITIONAL SUPPLEMENTS

In addition to the aforementioned supplements, there are other supplements that have been noted to benefit people with CKD when taken regularly. These include:

Vitamin E

Vitamin E is a great supplement for CKD. It can also help treat high blood pressure and a research study was conducted to evaluate the effects of high-dose vitamin E supplementation on markers of inflammation, urinary protein and oxidative stress in CKD patients with very positive results on all of the above. The recommended doses are 800 to 1200IU per day.

NOW Foods

395 S. Glen Ellyn Road

Bloomingdale, IL 60108

1-888-669-3663

www.nowfoods.com

Product: Vitamin E-400 Mixed Tocopherols - 100 Softgels. Take 1 pill two to three times per day.

Vitamin C

Vitamin C is a supplement long considered essential to boosting and maintaining a powerful immune system. In cases of kidney disease, Vitamin C can be beneficial if you're also suffering from anemia and is generally a very good antioxidant. Recommended dose is up to 1500mg per day in one or two divided doses.

American Health Sciences

2100 Smithtown Avenue

Ronkonkoma NY 11779

1-800-445-7137

Product: Ester-C purchase 500 or 1000mg with Citrus Bioflavonoids per capsule. Take 1000 to 1500mg per day in one to two divided doses.

N-A-C

N-A-C, which stands for n-acetyl-cysteine neutralizes toxins and pollutants including heavy metals that accumulate in the liver, kidneys, brain and fatty parts of the body. Restoring glutathione levels with NAC supplements makes liver cells more able to protect themselves from ongoing damage caused by fatty accumulation (fatty liver), viral infections, drug induced damage, alcohol excess or autoimmune inflammation. The recommended dose is 600-1000mg twice per day.

NOW Foods

395 S. Glen Ellyn Road

Bloomingdale, IL 60108

1-888-669-3663

www.nowfoods.com

Product: N-Acetyl-Cysteine 1000 mg, 120 Tablets

Take 1 pill twice per day

Cordyceps

According to recent research in CKD patients who were not currently undergoing dialysis, treatment with cordyceps significantly decreased serum creatinine levels, increased creatinine clearance and reduced levels of protein in the urine. The recommended dose is 1500mg two to three times per day. NOW Foods

395 S. Glen Ellyn Road

Bloomingdale, IL 60108

1-888-669-3663

www.nowfoods.com

Product: Cordyceps 750 mg Vegetarian Capsules

Take 2 pills two to three times per day

Benfotiamine

Another B vitamin, B1 in the form of Benfotiamine at a dose of 100 to 300mg

per dayhas shown to reduce proteinuria, reduce AGE, and improve oxidative stress

in diabetic kidney disease.

Life Extension Foundation

5990 North Federal Highway

Fort Lauderdale, FL 33308

1-800-544-4440

www.lef.org

Product: Benfotiamine with Thiamine, 100 mg, 120 vegetarian capsules

Take 1 pill two to three times per day.

CHAPTER 18 COMMONLY ASKED QUESTIONS ABOUT THE PROGRAM

This is too many pills and lifestyle changes to make. What should I do?

It is understandable that the supplement protocol can be difficult to implement and maintain. Especially, if you are not used to making lifestyle changes and taking supplements.If it feels like there are just too many pills, I recommendusing only the supplements for your specific condition and whatever you can from the core program. You can also contact us for email support.

What about side effects from the supplements?

Anything you put in your body can have a side effect. Supplements are no different. Unlike prescription medications, you generally don't have serious side effects from supplements and many have GRAS (Generally Recognized As Safe) status. The risk of side effects from properly manufactured supplements is very low. The rare amount of cases compared to prescription medications of having serious side effects are from adulterated and contaminated products, large amounts of overconsumption and rare genetic interactions with certain ingredients. The supplements listed in this program have shown excellent safety profiles with low risk of side effects.

As mentioned earlier, anything you put in your body can have a side effect. Supplements do have side effects, but more commonly along the lines of stomach upset/nausea, constipation, diarrhea, headaches, dizziness, increased heart rate, allergies and other non-serious side effects. To be cautious, you can start with half the amount for one to two weeks and gradually work your way up if the supplements are well-tolerated.

When beginning any health program, you should have before and after blood work and monitor your vital signs such as your blood pressure, heart rate, etc. This will allow you to monitor and determine whether or not any new symptoms you are feeling are because of the supplements.

How much can I drink?

In stages one and two of kidney disease, you will most likely be able to drink as much as you like. In stages 3 to 5 you may or may not be restricted in the amounts to drink. Allow your medical doctor to decide if you should be restricting fluids. As a general rule drink 8, eight-ounce glasses per day of water or herbal teas. Ideally, half your body weight in ounces of water per day is preferred.

Won't my cholesterol go up since the diet has

extra calories from fat?

No, your cholesterol shouldn't go up, actually it should go down. The reason for this is that you are consuming healthy poly- and monounsaturated fats which have been shown to lower cholesterol. It is the saturated animal fats, trans- and hydrogenated fats that raise cholesterol. You should still be having your cholesterol monitored every 3 to 6 months.

Blood Test to Monitor and Manage Diabetes

When you have kidney disease, you should be having your doctor check your hemoglobin A1C (HbA1c), a blood test for risk, diagnoses and management for diabetes every 3 to 12 months. The hemoglobin A1C provides an average of blood sugar over the past 3 to 4 months. The normal range for the hemoglobin A1C test is between 4% and 5.6%. Hemoglobin A1c levels between 5.7% and 6.4% indicate increased risk of diabetes, and levels of 6.5% or higher indicate diabetes.

Keeping track of this number will let you know how aggressive you need to be in preventing diabetes.

What happens if I develop gas or bloating, or don't feel well on the program?

If you are not used to taking supplements you may develop gas, bloating or stomach upset. This is harmless and will go away in a short amount of time. Your body has to get used to consumingsupplements.

You may want to begin by gradually taking supplements. You can start by taking smaller amounts of supplements and adding in the full amounts over a week to two weeks. This will allow adequate time for your body to adjust to the changes.

How come you recommend higher doses than what is listed on some of the supplement labels?

Supplement manufacturers will put a recommended dose on the bottle, but this may differ from what doses are used in scientific studies. The recommended doses provided are what have been used in studies to best benefit your kidneys. Using doses listed on the products may not provide you with a therapeutic effect. Use the recommended doses listed in this guide.

How long should I take supplements for?

Unless stated, supplements are taken for the long term. Just like medication for kidney disease is given for life, most supplements will need to be maintained for the long term to provide optimal benefits.

If I take higher doses of supplements will the process be better or faster?

No, in fact it may cause complications. The doses recommended are what have been used with a good safety profile.

Can I take the supplements with prescription medications?

Yes, you can take the supplements with medications as many of them have been studied in conjunction. When taking any supplements or medications there is always some degree of risk with side effects, no matter how safe a supplement or medication has been shown to be. You should monitor your blood sugar (if a diabetic), as well as your blood pressure and blood work to be aware of any changes, as medications may need to be adjusted.

How often should I have blood work done?

When first starting the program you should have your blood work conducted every 3 to 6 weeks. As time goes on you can space out your blood work to every 3 to 6 months. Monitoring blood work and any changes is important and should be done often.

When should I see results?

Most people will see results over the course of 4 to 12 weeks. You may see improvement in as little as 2 weeks, but your CKD may stabilize and in the following months you will see that there is no progression of the disease.

I am pregnant. Can I do this program?

If you are pregnant or nursing there are aspects of the program you can do, however you should contact us so a kidney coach can you review your specific situation and customize a plan for you.

Can children do the program?

The supplements can be used, but with adjustments of the doses based on the child-friendly formula.

How To Determine a Child's Dosage Formula Based on Body Weight

This is a more reliable method of children dose calculation and it bases the dosage on a given amount of supplement per pound or kilogram of body weight.

Note: Round off all body weights in kilograms to the nearest whole number. (2.2 lbs. per kilogram)

Example: Let's say the children dose of an herb is 10 mg/kg/24 hours. Calculate *the daily dose of this drug for a 44-pound child.*

Step 1. Convert 44 pounds to kilograms. 44 pounds divided by 2.2 pounds = 20 kilograms.

Step 2. Multiply the child's weight by the dose.

20 kg x 10 mg/kg = 200 mg/24 hrs. Therefore, give the child 200 mg, once a day.

CITATIONS & REFERENCES

This program is based upon over 1500 peer reviewed journal articles which gives it scientific credence in addition to my extensive experience working with thousands of people with kidney disease. In my first edition, the citations took up an additional 32 pages, which the majority of people never looked at or cared for. Plus, it raises the price of the program due to the added cost of printing additional pages.

If you are interested in any citations and reference materials please contact us and what exactly you are interested in. Most major medical data in the United States with peer reviewed studies from around the world is catalogued in http://www.pubmed.com This is free to the public and by searching the information provided here you will most likely find the studies using human subjects.

FINAL THOUGHTS

Dealing with and managing your kidney disease is not an easy thing and something that should be taken seriously. This program gives you the options at your disposal to begin actively helping your kidney health. You choose what supplements you will be taking. You should take all your prescription medication as prescribed.

Diet is absolutely crucial for kidney disease. The kidney controls so many aspects of proper nutrition that diet plays a key role in improving kidney health. For dietary recommendations see our book called, "The Complete Guide To Renal Diet Plans & Cook Books" available on Amazonand our website: HealthyKidneyInc.com.

Using one approach to improving your kidney health ensures a lower chance of success. Using both approaches together will maximize your chances of supporting normal kidney function.

If you have any questions or would like personal coaching that is included with this program please contact us. healthykidneyinc@gmail.com

To Your Best Kidney Health,

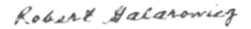

Made in the USA
Monee, IL
28 August 2020

40300310R00066